Lizbeth Olguín García

CT Gate in patients with CVD

Lizbeth Olguín García

CT Gate in patients with CVD

Mean CT door time in patients with a clinical diagnosis of CVE.

ScienciaScripts

Cover image: www.ingimage.com

This book is a translation from the original published under ISBN 978-613-9-40637-1.

Publisher:
Sciencia Scripts
is a trademark of
Dodo Books Indian Ocean Ltd. and OmniScriptum S.R.L publishing group

120 High Road, East Finchley, London, N2 9ED, United Kingdom
Str. Armeneasca 28/1, office 1, Chisinau MD-2012, Republic of Moldova, Europe
Managing Directors: Ieva Konstantinova, Victoria Ursu
info@omniscriptum.com

Printed at: see last page
ISBN: 978-620-8-50894-4

INDEX

ACKNOWLEDGEMENTS 3

INTRODUCTION 6

THEORETICAL FRAMEWORK 9

METHODOLOGY 22

RESULTS 23

DISCUSSION...29

CONCLUSION AND RECOMMENDATION......................36

REFERENCES...37

DEDICATION

To my mother for her endless love and unconditional support. To my daughter Ellis, for being the inspiration and motivation of my days.

ACKNOWLEDGEMENTS

To my advisors for this content, Dr. Rigoberto Martínez Parroquin, Dr. Leoncio Miguel Rodríguez Guzmán and Dr. Ilsia Vinalay Carrillo for always instructing and motivating me in this research.

MEAN CT DOOR TIME IN PATIENTS WITH A CLINICAL DIAGNOSIS OF CVD

SUMMARY

Introduction: *Cerebral vascular event (CVE) is the second leading cause of death worldwide, where two thirds are of ischaemic origin, causing disability, therefore, some health institutions have made proposals to establish timely diagnosis and treatment.* ***Objective: To*** *describe adherence to the Comprehensive Care Protocol-Brain Code (PAI brain code) in a second level care unit.* ***Methods:*** *A cross-sectional, descriptive study was conducted in a second-level hospital in Minatitlán, Veracruz. Thirty patients with a clinical diagnosis of CVE were included and the following variables were measured: age, sex, types of CVE, comorbidities, time to the tomographic study and time in the care process, as well as patient follow-up during the first 7 days of the event.* ***Results:*** *The mean age was 66.2 ±, 15.6 (28 - 91) years. The majority of cases were male (63.3%). Mean medical and nursing assessment time was 0.84±, 0.78 (0.10 - 3) hours and door time had a mean of 39.04 ± 41.01 (2 - 192) hours.* ***Conclusion:*** *100% of the patients did not comply with the time established by the PAI Brain Code.*

Keywords*: Cerebral infarction; cerebral haemorrhage; essential hypertension; cerebral ischaemia*

INTRODUCTION

CVE is characterised by acute neurological dysfunction that can last more than 24 hours and lead to death. There are two main types of CVE depending on the aetiology: ischaemic resulting from occlusion of the blood vessel to or within the brain due to thrombus or embolus formation and haemorrhagic resulting from rupture of an artery within (intracerebral haemorrhage) or on the surface (subarachnoid haemorrhage) of the brain (López Tapia et al., 2022).

Worldwide it is the second cause of death and the leading cause of disability in adults, with an incidence of 190 cases per 100 000 inhabitants each year, of which 44% have a functional dependence and 90% remain with sequelae. In INEGI statistics for 2019, 35 303 deaths were recorded and by 2030 an increase of 44% and a disability of 200 million individuals is expected. In the Mexican Social Security Institute (IMSS) it has been categorised as one of the 10 main chronic diseases (PAI Código cerebro, 2022).

There are risk factors associated with CVE, both non-modifiable (age, sex and genetic factors) and modifiable (systemic arterial hypertension, obesity, increased apolipoprotein B, dyslipidaemia, smoking, diabetes mellitus). Obesity and arterial hypertension are the most prevalent (García González et al., 2022), with a greater distribution in men (Choreño Parra et al., 2019).

Symptoms associated with BSS are related to sudden-onset motor weakness, which may or may not be transient, in one or more body segments (face, arm, hand, leg), sudden-onset dysphasia with sensory loss in 2 or more body segments, sudden-onset hemianopsia or quadrantanopsia with transient visual loss in part of the visual field (hemianopsia homonymous or quadrantanopsia), sudden onset monocular vision loss of transient monocular visual loss, as well as vertigo, diplopia, dysarthria and ataxia (Tuna and Rothwell, 2021).

The initial clinical diagnosis is made in first level units or triage areas of emergency departments Calero Moscoso, 2023). In the latter areas, some institutions apply prognostic scales such as the Cincinnati scale, which estimates an 89% probability of CVE; the prognostic percentage decreases according to the clinical characteristics foundfor example, if only one sign is found, the probability decreases to 72% (Mohamed et al., 2022). Another scale for assessing neurological deficit is the well-known NIHSS (National Institute of Health Stroke Scale), which is used to determine the most appropriate treatment, predict outcome and short- and long-term prognosis (Ali Khan et al., 2022).

Diagnostic imaging by plain skull tomography is considered the imaging study of choice for CVE (Edzie et al., 2021), indicated within the first 25 minutes of symptom onset, with a sensitivity in the first 6 hours of 39% and a specificity of 94% (PAI Brain Code, 2022), when identifying cerebral ischaemic changes, the ASPECTS tomographic scale is applied to predict the functional prognosis and risk of cerebral haemorrhage in patients with ischaemic CVE or to determine whether it is haemorrhagic CVE or normal brain tissue; consists of 10 points, and each region with ischaemic changes equals 1 point (Phipps and Cronin, 2020), a score of> 8 points is considered optimal for fibrinolytic therapy, a score equal to or less than 7 points rules out fibrinolysis (PAI Brain Code, 2022).

Globally, there are improvement processes for early diagnosis and treatment, such as the PAI Brain Code programme. The aim of this programme is to The aim of the programme is to standardise the actions of medical staff at the first, second and third levels of care in the management of people with CVE. One of its indicators is timely treatment based on intravenous fibrinolytic therapy within the first 60 minutes of admission to the emergency department, preventing and treating complications in the first 24 to 72 hours of CVE, implementing early rehabilitation from the first 48 hours and, in the long term, stratifying the risk of recurrence of CVE before discharge, all contribute to reducing morbidity and mortality and achieving the well-being of the beneficiaries; It has been shown that patients admitted to a hospital unit with a specialised multidisciplinary BSS team have shorter hospital days, better prognosis and physical dependency than those units that do not (PAI Brain Code, 2022).

Since there are few up-to-date studies on compliance with the brain code indicators, the aim of the present study was to describe the behaviour of these indicators in a second-level care unit.

THEORETICAL FRAMEWORK

The cerebral vascular event is due to disorders that compromise the cerebral vasculature and produce a decrease in cerebral blood flow resulting in cerebral damage, which may be transient or permanent, and may occur in a generalised or focal manner, with no apparent cause other than vascular origin. It can be further subdivided into: Established vascular event where the neurological deficit persists and lasts more than three weeks from its onset, leaving the patient with neurological sequelae, Stable vascular event: the neurological deficit persists unchanged for 24 hours (in cases of carotid origin) or 72 hours (in cases of vertebrobasilar origin), then evolves into a reversible neurological deficit or an established vascular event, and into an evolving vascular event: the neurological deficit increases and the picture worsens or new symptoms appear within 24 to 48 hours (López Tapia et al, 2022). Factors associated with haemorrhagic vascular event include the following: Uncontrolled high blood pressure, overtreatment with anticoagulants, Aneurysms and arteriovenous malformations, trauma, cerebral amyloid angiopathy, ischaemic vascular event with haemorrhagic conversion. They are most often divided into two groups according to the mechanism, usually ischaemic or haemorrhagic: Ischaemic (85% of cases): Thrombotic: Lacunar infarction: occlusion of small cerebral vessels occluding the blood supply to a small volume of brain tissue, Infarction of a large blood vessel. Embolic: Cardioembolic: the embolism comes from the heart, often from the left atrium, Artery-artery, Cryptogenic: the occlusion of an intracranial vessel without apparent cause - Haemorrhagic: Intraparenchymal, Subdural, Epidural, Subarachnoid (López Tapia et al, 2022).The cerebral circulation is supplied by the carotid arteries (which provide about 80% of total cerebral perfusion) and the vertebral arteries. The right common carotid artery emerges from the brachiocephalic trunk, the first branch of the aortic arch, while the left common carotid artery is a direct branch of the arch. In the neck, it divides into the internal and external carotids, ending its medial course at the anterior clinoid process, where it divides into 3 branches important for the cerebral circulation: anterior, middle and posterior communicating cerebral artery, thus forming the anterior circulation. Between 0.5 and 3% of ischaemic cerebral vascular accidents occur in the territory of the anterior cerebral artery, 5 to 10% in that of the posterior cerebral artery and 50-80% occur in the territory the middle cerebral artery (Pineda and Tolosa, 2022).

The middle cerebral artery is the most common artery involved in acute stroke. These vessels provide blood supply to parts of the frontal, temporal and parietal lobes of the brain, as well as to deeper structures, including the caudate, internal capsule and thalamus (Nogles and Galuska, 2022).

After an acute ischaemic stroke, the inflammatory process evolves in three stages: The acute phase in the first hours after stroke onset, during which microglia/macrophages clear necrotic cells and a first influx of leukocytes, mainly neutrophils, has been described. The subacute phase during the first days after the ischaemic insult, associated with a resolution of the inflammatory process and the late phase, in which inflammatory cells contribute to astrocytic and microglial reparative processes (Jurcau and Simion, 2021). The expected symptoms in a patient with a cerebral vascular event are: Sudden-onset, transient motor weakness in one or more segments of the brain. body (face, arm, hand, leg). Onset dysphasia with sensory loss in two or more body segments (face, arm, hand or leg). Sudden onset hemianopsia or quadrantanopsia with transient visual loss in part of the visual field (homonymous hemianopsia or quadrantanopsia). Sudden onset monocular vision loss with transient monocular visual loss. Vertigo, diplopia, dysarthria and ataxia (Tuna and Rothwell, 2021).Single skull tomography is the imaging study of choice for cerebral vascular events, able to accurately diagnose and distinguish between ischaemic and haemorrhagic stroke. The acute and chronic phase that can develop after a stroke sequence is clearly defined by CT despite many improvements in MRI technology, and is the most widely used for assessment due to its rapid image acquisition and availability in most radiological practices (Edzie et al, 2021).

Its sensitivity to haemorrhage, rapid acquisition and wide availability make it the ideal first study. Computed tomography angiography, the most common follow-up study after non-contrast head CT, is primarily used to identify large intracranial vessel occlusions and cervical or vertebral carotid artery disease. CT angiography is very sensitive and can improve the accuracy of patient selection for endovascular therapy through ischaemic core delineations. Magnetic resonance imaging and magnetic resonance angiography can provide valuable information for prognostic outcome as well as stroke aetiology (Czap and Sheth, 2021). The basal ganglia area, which lies under the territory of the middle cerebral artery, is the most common anatomical location of stroke events in our environment, followed by the parietal lobe and then the frontal lobe. Knowing the anatomical locations of these stroke events has an impact on the type of management needed, especially in the early of these events. Men suffer significantly more strokes in the basal ganglia, while strokes located in the pons were more frequently observed in women (Hadijat et al, 2020).

There are two main therapies for ischaemic stroke: thrombolysis and thrombectomy. However, their applications in clinical practice are still very limited due to the short treatment window (Bao et al, 2022). Fibrinolytic, anticoagulant and antiplatelet drugs are the three main options to combat thrombotic diseases, working through the respective removal of the fibrin network, inhibition of the coagulation cascade and platelet activation (Xu et al, 2021).Tissue plasminogen activator (rTPA) is an intravenous drug that works by enhancing the conversion of inactive plasminogen to active plasmin, which in turn causes lysis of fibrin clots with the of restoring cerebral blood perfusion (Coronel et al, 2020).

Indications Absolute contraindications Relative contraindications

– Over 18 years old

- Diagnosis of HF causing the neurological deficit

- Symptom onset less than 4.5 hours

- Signing of informed consent

– CT scan shows multilobar infarction (hypodensity > cerebral hemisphere).

– Head trauma or BSS in previous 3 months

– Cranial or spinal surgery within the previous 3 months

– Symptoms suggestive of subarachnoid haemorrhage

– Seizure at onset and suspicion of residual deficit

– Minor and isolated symptoms (NIHSS* less than 4

– Systolic blood pressure> 185 mmHg and diastolic

>110 mmHg persistent

– History of previous cerebral haemorrhage

– Evidence of active bleeding or active trauma on physical examination

– Taking oral anticoagulants with INR greater than 1.

– If used heparin in previous 48 hours, abnormal TTP

– Platelets less than 100 000/mm3

– Glucose less than 50 mg/dL and greater than 400 mg/dL

– Arterial puncture at non-compressive site on previous seven days

– Factor Xa inhibitor use in the last 4 hours

- Symptoms are spontaneously subsiding in moderate myocardial infarction.

– Major surgery 14 days prior

- Acute myocardial infarction 3 months earlier

– Pregnancy

- Gastrointestinal or urinary bleeding within the previous 21 days

– Major head trauma in the last 14 days

- Suspected arterial dissection

– Suspected endocarditis

– Malignant intracranial neoplasm, art bacterial malformation

venous or cerebral aneurysm

– Acute pancreatitis

– Age over 80 years

– NIHSS scale greater than 25

Endovascular therapy (EVT)

Indications

-Less than 6 hours of evolution

– Over 18 years old

– NIHSS scale greater than 6 points (moderate to severe)

– Pre-CSE Rankin Scale less than 2 (adequate functional status prior to CSE).

– ASPECT scale greater than 6 (moderate infarction by imaging)

– Proximal artery occlusion demonstrated by angio-tomography or angio-resonance angiography

FIBRINOLYTIC THERAPY

Table 1. Indications and contraindications for fibrinolytic therapy.

Fármac

o Acetylsalicylic acid li-cyl acid

	Start 24 hours after BSS	Suspend 7 days prior to surgery program me da	80 a 325 mg/day	Hypersensitivity to the drug, active peptic ulcer or gastritis, hypoprothrombinemia.	Prolonged bleeding time, tinnitus, hearing loss, nausea, vomiting, gastrointestinal bleeding, hepatitis, ecchymosis, ecchymosis, rash, asthma, hypersensitivity reactions
	Start 24 hours after BSS	Discontinue 7 days before surgery day program	150mg loading dose, continuous r 75 mg every 24 hours	Hypersensitivity to the drug, active bleeding and liver failure.	Diarrhoea, gastrointestinal bleeding, thrombocytopenia
	3-4 days up to INR optimal.	Depends on INR control in range.	Start on the 4th to 7th day in EVC cardioe	Hypersensitivity to the drug, lactation, tuberculosis, active bleeding.	Increased serum transaminases, haemorrhage. Start of action Duration of effect Dosage ContraindicationsAdverse effect Clopido-grel Aceno- cumarina

mbolic .INR target 2.5-3.5				
At	24hrs.	20 mg	Hypersensitivity to	Hepatopathy, increased
24hrs		oral	drug and patients	DHL and alkaline phosphatase,
		each	with bleeding	dizziness, headache, syncope,
		24hrs	active, clinically	renal failure, pruritus,
		in BSS	significant, such as	rash, urticaria,
		cardioe	haemorrhage	haemorrhage
		mbolic	intracranial,	after intervention,
		with	haemorrhage	tube haemorrhage
		contrain	digestive system,	digestive and digestive system
		dication	Renal insufficiency.	reproductive, haematuria,
		for		epistaxis
		acenocu		
		marine.		
1-2	14 hours	40-80	Hypersensitivity to	Discomfort
hours		mg/dl	drug, pregnancy,	gastrointestinal,
			breastfeeding and	headache, myalgia, asthenia,
			disease	insomnia.
			active liver,	
			kidney failure	
			at	
			treatment	
			substitute	Rivaro- xaban Atorvas -tatina

Source: Brain Code Working Group, 2020

In Mexico, the reported cases of successful thrombolysis are only 5%. In this successful case, the appropriate action in the first contact Emergency Department had a positive impact on the patient's prognosis, as the timely diagnosis and administration of rTPA (tissue plasminogen activator) prevented important sequelae and achieved a better quality of life, which is diminished in up to 70% of patients who suffer a cerebral vascular event (Romero et al, 2018). Mechanical thrombectomy has been shown to be associated with improved functional outcomes for patients with ischaemic stroke. acute with proximal anterior circulation, large vessel occlusion and salvageable brain tissue (Almallouhi et al, 2021).Brain haemorrhages have various causes, such as traumatic brain injury, hypertension or intracranial tumours. In general, they are usually divided into five types of haemorrhages, depending mainly on the area where they occur: Epidural Haemorrhage, Subdural Haemorrhage, Subarachnoid Haemorrhage, Intracerebral Haemorrhage and Intraventricular Haemorrhage (Solorio et al, 2021).

Neurosurgical treatment may be considered in patients with supratentorial intracranial haemorrhage who present with neurological deterioration, coma, significant midline deviation or elevated intracranial pressure refractory to medical treatment. The aim is to decompress the brain and reduce the impact of mass effect, malignant oedema and toxic blood by-products (Man et al, 2021).

The initial assessment of a patient with evidence of neurological alteration should be carried out at first contact in the triage area, where the preliminary clinical assessment process is carried out, which allows the patient's need for medical attention to be prioritised and classified, with five classes (colours) of patients according to the seriousness of the reason for medical attention: resuscitation, emergency, urgency, minor urgency and no urgency. Priority is given to real or true emergencies. Needle-door time: the time from the onset of symptoms of a cerebral vascular event to the initiation of fibrinolytic therapy (Phipps and Cronin, 2020).

Acute ischaemic stroke and intracerebral haemorrhage cannot be distinguished clinically, and thrombolytic therapy is effective in the former and detrimental to the latter. , all patients with a suspected ischaemic vascular event, a non-contrast CT scan of the head should be performed for initial management. The CT scan should be performed within 20 minutes of the patient's arrival. If it does not delay intravenous thrombolysis, non-invasive intracranial vascular imaging should be performed in patients who meet the criteria for endovascular clot retrieval. For early ischaemic changes on computed tomography, the ASPECTS Score has been used; it is a semi-quantitative tomographic scale developed to optimise the identification of cerebral ischaemic changes in the three-hour window of intravenous thrombolysis with recombinant tissue plasminogen activator. It predicts functional prognosis and risk of cerebral haemorrhage. The ASPECT tomographic scale evaluates ischaemic changes in territory of the anterior cerebral circulation, it consists of 10 points, for each region showing ischaemic changes one point is decreased, the higher the score the higher the degree of cerebral ischaemia (Phipps and Cronin, 2020).

Scales exist for identifying the patient and getting them to the correct treatment more quickly, the National Institutes of Health Stroke Scale (NIHSS), Los Angeles Motor Scale (LAMS), Vision, Aphasia and Neglect (VAN) screening tool had the best predictive value for early detection (Phipps and Cronin, 2020).

Other scales to be performed upon arrival at prehospital triage: the 3-item stroke scale (3I-SS), Cincinnati Prehospital Stroke Severity Scale, FAST, Texas Stroke Intervention Prehospital Stroke Severity Scale, Melbourne Ambulance Stroke Screen, Medic Prehospital Assessment for Code Stroke, Ontario Prehospital Stroke Screening, RACE and ROSIER (Teleb et al, 2017). The Cincinnati Prehospital Stroke Scale with a score of 3, assessing facial asymmetry, arm descent and abnormal speech, is an easy and reliable screening tool to classify patients with ischaemic stroke and large vessel occlusion, without going through a primary stroke centre, without significantly increasing the frequency of stroke mimics (Mohamed et al, 2022). The National Institute of Health Stroke Scale (NIHSS) is a scale for quantitative assessment of neurological deficit after acute cerebral vascular accident, used to measure the deterioration of patients with CVA, determine the most appropriate examinations and treatment, and predict the patient's evolution; it is a short- and long-term prognostic tool (Ali et al, 2022).The Los Angeles Motor Scale (LAMS): belonging to the most predictive scale, requiring the assessment of only three motor symptoms (facial paresis, arm strength and grip strength), the following factors were considered: 1. LAMS score (cut-off score of 4); 2. symptom onset times of 8 h or less or presence of stroke 3. quality of life aspects, such as severe comorbid conditions and severe dependency prior to stroke (Behnke et al, 2021).

The vision, aphasia and neglect assessment scale for stroke with large vessel occlusion: this was initially tested in a small study where emergency department (ED) nurses were trained to perform VAN assessment in stroke code patients (Navalkele et al, 2020). Clinical diagnosis of cerebral infarction on arrival at triage: Recognition of the symptoms and signs of the disease, applying the Cincinnati scale. If any of the three clinical signs is abnormal (facial asymmetry, lowering of the arm or altered language), the probability of CVE is 72%, if all three signs are altered the probability increases to 89%. Because of the importance of the time of symptom onset, the following is recommended: If the time of symptom onset is unclear, start counting from the last time the patient was observed as normal. If the patient woke up with signs or symptoms, start counting from the time he/she went to sleep. If the symptoms are intermittent, start counting from the last time they started. Question in a targeted manner about cardiovascular risk factors and ask for a history of trauma or surgery, recent or active gastrointestinal or urinary bleeding, or active history of bleeding that contraindicates TF. When the patient is stabilised, a rapid general and neurological examination should be performed to look for alterations in mental functions, cranial nerves, muscle strength, sensation or cerebellum. Patients with confusional state without focal disturbances or who present with isolated vertigo or headache have a low probability of CVE. Identify poor prognostic clinical features such as: coma, gaze deviation, verbal unresponsiveness and severe midbody weakness, clinically indicative of extensive infarction. In these cases, intravenous TF is contraindicated. It is important to make a differential diagnosis with clinical history and tomography, to rule out pathologies simulating cerebral infarction (intracranial haemorrhage, neoplasms of the nervous system, hypoglycaemia, convulsive crises, psychiatric disorders, among others) (PAI Brain Code, 2022). Diagnostic imaging of cerebral infarction. A simple cranial CT scan is essential to rule out haemorrhagic stroke before giving a diagnosis of cerebral infarction. TF to a patient, its sensitivity for Cerebral Infarction in the first 6 hours is 39% and specificity is 94%, thus allowing the diagnosis of IH to be ruled out. CT perfusion and MRI are more sensitive and are recommended if available, but should not delay initiation of treatment. In patients with a clinical diagnosis of HF, CT should be performed in less than 25 minutes to rule out IH and with the ASPECT scale to assess the severity of HF (Scale 5), if it is> 8 points should be considered for TF. An ASPECT scale equal to or less than 7 points indicates an extensive infarction and TF should be avoided. As well as the presence of IH, old haemorrhages or other structural alteration that explains the patient's symptoms (PAI Brain Code, 2022). Poor prognostic tomographic findings (early signs extensive HF and contraindication of TF: 1. Hyperdense MCA sign (A) 2. 3. Erasure of the insula. 4. Erasure of the sulci of more than one third of the cerebral hemisphere (B). 5. loss of differentiation between grey matter and white matter in more than one third of the middle cerebral artery territory (B) (PAI Brain Code, 2022). Treatment with fibrinolytic therapy (FFT) in patients with cerebral infarction. The approved drug used and available at the institute for TF is Alteplase. It is important to take into consideration the following: 1. The door-to-needle time should be less than 60 minutes (each optimised minute correlates with less residual disability). 2. The results of laboratory or special studies should not delay the start of treatment. 3. In patients with a history of treatment with oral anticoagulants, suspected thrombocytopenia or coagulation disorder, blood biometry for platelet count or clotting times, as appropriateshould be performed beforehand. 4. Monitor closely during TF administration, discontinue drug infusion immediately and perform urgent CT scan of the skull if the patient has a history of thrombocytopenia. the following serious warning signs and symptoms: Anaphylactic reaction. Severe (severe) headache. Increase of 4 points on the NIHSS scale. Deterioration of alertness. The patient should remain under close surveillance during the first 24 hours of TF onset, BP monitoring every 15 minutes for the first hour and then every 30 minutes for the next 5 hours, thereafter, the frequency is hourly for 24 hours. In case of SBP> 180 or DBP > 105 mmHg increase monitoring frequency and administer parenteral antihypertensives. In case of arterial hypotension, administer vasopressors to maintain cerebral perfusion pressure at target levels. 6. 24 hours after the administration of TF, it is recommended that a simple phase cranial CT scan be performed prior to the indication of antiplatelet agents (PAI Brain Code, 2022). Adjuvant treatment and control goals should be focused on restoring cerebral blood flow and minimising the infarct zone, so primary measures are based on head position at 30 degrees for the first 48 hours, Maintain Cerebral Perfusion Pressure greater than 65 mmHg. The brain has its own self-regulating mechanisms with a limit of 60 to 180 mmHg, Maintain oxygenation with SpO2 > 94%, Maintain paCO2 levels between 35 and 40 mmHg. In case of severe cerebral oedema maintain between 30 and 35 mmHg (only as an intermediate measure as the effect lasts for a few minutes), Fluid management with adequate intravascular volume using isotonic solution such as sodium chloride 0.9% sodium chloride at 30 ml/kg body weight, with a target central venous pressure of 5 to 10 mmHg; avoid overload, Indicate antiepileptics only if seizures are present (not indicated as a preventive measure), Temperature: physical means and paracetamol 500 to 1000 mg every 8 hours if> 37.5ºC, Blood glucose every

2-4 hours: Treat blood glucose values > 180 mg/dl with insulin and correcting hypoglycaemia (< 50 mg/dl) with dextroseIntravenous or 10-20% glucose infusion, Perform intubation for mechanical ventilation if the patient presents respiratory compromise or Glasgow Coma Scale of less than 8, Evaluation of dysphagia and bronchoaspiration, assess tube placement prior to TF but without delaying the time of administration, Prevent the development of cerebral oedema: avoid hypo-osmolar solutions, hyperthermia, hypoxia, hypercapnia. If oedema causes neurological deterioration, start treatment with mannitol or hyperosmolar solutions, Start diet ideally between the 2nd and 4th day, after swallowing test and nutritional assessment, Avoid as far as possible drugs that depress the central nervous system (neuroleptics, benzodiazepines, barbiturates), prevention, prevention, surveillance and early treatment of healthcare-associated infections, prevention of venous thrombosis with the use of elastic bandages and subcutaneous enoxaparin, mobilisation of the patient according to clinical condition and risk scale for pressure ulcers, gastric protection with omeprazole, early physical rehabilitation if there are no contraindications (PAI Brain Code, 2022). The prognosis for life and the reduction of neurological sequelae following a cerebral vascular event can be improved with comprehensive care plans. Older age, female gender, lower educational level, greater disability, anxiety and depression are associated with poor quality of life, and failure to conduct accurate and adequate questioning will have an impact on the functional dependence of patients suffering from a cerebral vascular event (Orman et al, 2022).

METHODOLOGY

This book describes how an observational, descriptive, prospective, descriptive study was carried out, including all patients who attended the emergency department between October 2023 and March 2024, men and women over 20 years of age. The sample size was 30 patients to whom the NIHSS and Cincinnati prehospital scales were applied to gather the probable diagnosis score of CVE, subsequently confirmed with a cranial CT scan. All patients and responsible relatives agreed to participate in the study by means of informed consent; those with other pathologies of neurological origin were excluded. The variables studied were age, sex, types of CVE, comorbidities, time prior to the tomographic study and times in the care process, as well as patient follow-up during the first 7 days after the event. An instrument was applied and its content evaluated by an emergency physician, an epidemiologist and a family physician. Statistical analysis was performed using SPSS version 25, where simple and absolute frequencies, mean and standard deviation were obtained.

RESULTS

The total sample size of the study was 30 patients; mean age was 66.17 ±, 15.545 (28 - 91) years. In relation to sex 19 (63.3%) were male and 11 (36.7%) were female. Smoking was identified as a cause of cardiovascular risk in six (20%) patients, alcohol consumption in three (10%) patients and sedentary lifestyle in 30 (100%) patients. Of the comorbidities associated with CVD, systemic arterial hypertension in 23 (76.7%) patients was the main related disease, followed by type 2 diabetes mellitus in 18 (60%) patients, dyslipidaemia in 14 (46.7%) patients, heart disease in three (10%) patients, arrhythmias in two (6.7%) patients, and a history of CVD in six (20%) patients.

Table 1. Distribution of anthropometric grades according to BMI

Grades	Frequency	Percentage
Underweight	1	3.3 %
Normal weight	12	40 %
Overweight	9	30 %
Obesity Grade I	4	13.3 %
Obesity Grade ll	3	10 %
Obesity Grade III	1	3.3%

In the results obtained for BMI, the highest percentage in relation to weight was normal weight in 12 (40%) patients, followed by overweight in nine (30%) patients.

Figure 1. Cincinnati Scale

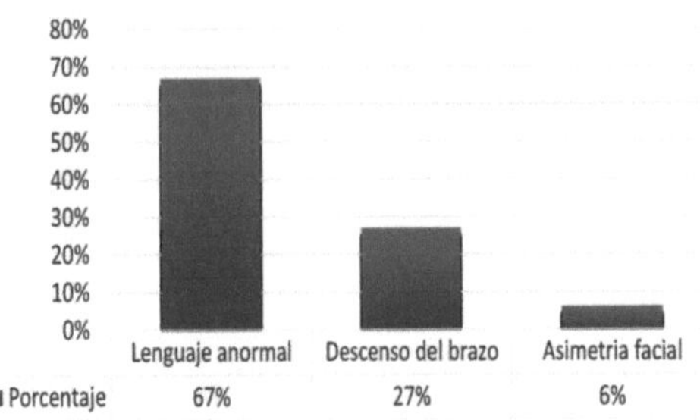

According to the Cincinnati scale the 86% chance of CVE was found in 19 (63.3%) patients, 73-85% chance of CVE in eight (26.7%) patients and 72% chance of CVE in two (6.7%) patients.

Table 2. NIHSS Neurological Assessment Scale

NIHSS	Day 1	Day 2	Day 3	Day 4	Day 5	Day 6	Day 7
Slight	2	2	3	3	4	5	4
Mild to moderate	9	8	5	7	8	9	9
Moderate to serious	14	15	18	17	13	9	9
Very serious	5	5	3	2	2	2	2
Expenditure	0	0	1	1	3	5	6

The NIHSS scale found that moderate to severe BSS (11-20 points) occurred in 14 (46.7%) patients, mild to moderate BSS (5-10 points) in nine patients, and mild to moderate BSS (5-10 points) in four patients, and moderate to severe BSS (5-10 points) in four patients, and mild to moderate BSS (5-10 points) in four patients. (30%) patients. Day 3 was determined to be the most critical, as an increase in the neurological assessment scale was obtained, finding moderate to severe NIHSS in 18 (60%) patients, with a decrease on days 6 and 7 with moderate to severe NIHSS in only nine (30%) patients, and mild to moderate in nine (30%) patients. Simple cranial CT found a diagnosis of ischaemic stroke in 24 (80%) patients, haemorrhagic stroke in five (16.7%) patients, and transient cerebral ischaemia in one (3.3%) patient.

Figure 2. ASPECT Quantitative Tomography Scale

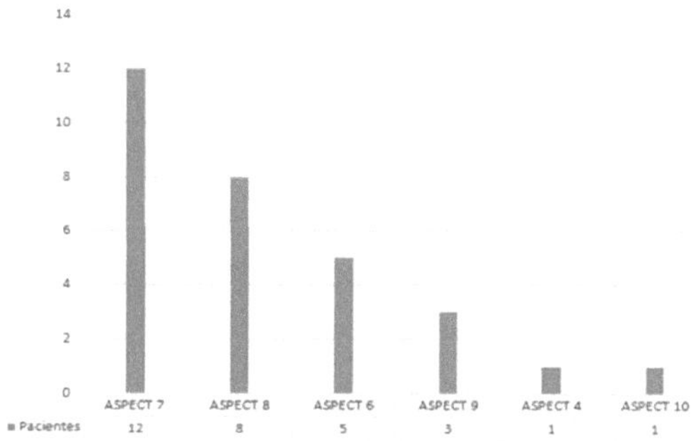

	ASPECT 7	ASPECT 8	ASPECT 6	ASPECT 9	ASPECT 4	ASPECT 10
■ Pacientes	12	8	5	3	1	1

When applying the ASPECT tomographic scale where ischaemic changes in the anterior cerebral circulation were assessed we found that the most frequent score was 7 in 12 (40%) patients, followed by a score of 8 in eight (26.7%) patients and a score of 6 in four (16.7%) patients. As for the initial medical care at first contact, it was carried out by the general practitioner with a frequency of 15 (50%) patients, followed by the doctor. emergency physician in 13 (43.3%) patients and family physician in two (6.7%) patients. In the assessment by specialties from initial care, by internal medicine service, it was performed in 30 (100%) patients, with the earliest assessment at 3 hours in one (3.3%) patient and the latest at 96 hours in one (3.3%) patient. Neurological assessment was carried out in five (16.7%) patients, the earliest being at 15 hours in one (3.3%) patient and the latest at 48 hours in one 3.3%) patient. Four (13.3%) patients were assessed by the speciality of neurosurgery, with early attention at 72 hours in one (3.3%) patient and late at 120 hours in one (3.3%) patient.

In relation to clinical/diagnostic and treatment congruence according to the PAI brain code, the corresponding antihypertensive drugs were not used in 30 (100%) patients. However, other types of antihypertensives were used in 12 patients where the most frequent use was the combination of ARA II plus Calcium antagonists in four (13.3%) patients, as single antihypertensive ACE inhibitors in four (13.3%) patients, ARA II in three (10%) patients and Calcium antagonists in one (3.3%) patient. Antiplatelet therapy was managed with ASA in 11 (36.7%) patients and Clopidogrel in 16 (53.3%) patients. In statin therapy Atorvastatin was used in 24 (80%) patients. Adherence to the criteria of the PAI code brain in all 30 (100%) patients, none of them applied the stipulations of the algorithm.

Table 3. Approach time in the emergency department for patients with VTE

	Brain code	Minimum Time	Maximum Time
Immediate entry	0-5 minutes	22 minutes	96 hours
Medical assessment and nursing	0-10 minutes	10 minutes	3 hours
Imaging	0-25 minutes	2 hours	192 hours

In terms of patient arrival time at the emergency department for initial care, the mean time was 21.10 ± 25.62 (0.22 - 96) hours. Medical and nursing assessment with a mean time of 0.84± 0.78 (0.10 - 3) hours. Cranial CT had a mean time of 39.04± 41.01 (2 - 192) hours. According to the times found, the evaluation and administration of thrombolysis is outside the window. We found that 28 (93.3%) patients presented with sequelae following CVE, with dysarthria occurring most frequently in 27 (90%) patients, facial paralysis in 23 (76.7%) patients, and hemiplegia in 18 (60%) patients, Broca's aphasia in 14 (46.7%) patients, haemiparesis in 12 (40%) patients patients, dysphagia in 8 (26.7%) patients, spasticity in 5 (16.7%) patients, loss of balance in 5 (16.7%) patients, seizures in

3 (10%) patients, Wernicke's aphasia in 2 (6.7%) patients, incontinence in 2 (6.7%) patients, and incontinence in 3 (10%) patients. 2 (6.7%) patients. In the 3-month follow-up of the evolution of the sequelae, we found 4 subgroups of patients after CVE.

Figure 3. Patient subgroups post-CSE

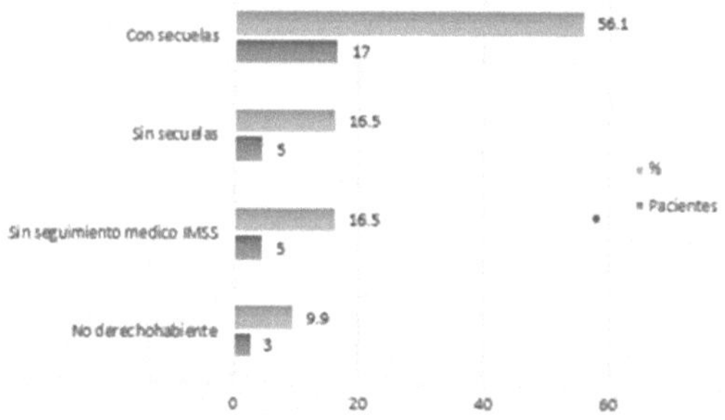

Five (16.5%) patients did not continue treatment and follow-up at the , as they opted to continue private management, while other patients lost their hospital registration during follow-up, three (9.9%) of them.

Table 4. Percentage of sequelae occurring within 3 months of BSS.

Sequel	Patients	%
Dysarthria	9	29.7
Dyslalia	1	3.3
Dysphagia	2	6.6
Aphasia	5	16.5
Hemiplegia	9	29.7
Hemiparesis	1	3.3
Erectile dysfunction	1	3.3
Urinary incontinence	1	3.3
Seizures	2	6.6
Spasticity	3	9.9
Facial paralysis	7	13.2

In one of the subgroups, represented by 17 (56.1%) patients, we found that dysarthria and hemiplegia persisted in nine (29.7%) patients, while facial paralysis persisted in 7 (13.2%) patients. In addition, there are patients who remain functionally dependent, of which cane use is represented in 2 (6.6%) patients, wheelchair support in 3 (9.9%) patients and urinary incontinence with Foley catheter use in one (3.3%) patient. We also observed that there are patients who, despite management by physical medicine and rehabilitation together with the internal medicine specialty, were not able to reintegrate to their daily activities. In this subgroup of 17 patients, four (13.2%) patients applied for a pension, two (6.6%) patients returned to work, three (9.9%) patients were temporarily incapacitated, one (3.3%) patient was unemployed, and two (6.6%) patients died within three months despite medical follow-up.

DISCUSSION

CVE is considered to be a neurological emergency, worldwide every year around 6 million people die; it is caused by the loss of balance between oxygen supply and consumption (Figueroa Casanova et al., 2022), 80% of its aetiology is of ischaemic origin, of thrombotic, embolic or haemodynamic cause, causing brain damage, transient or permanent and generalised or focal (López Tapia et al., 2022).In a study conducted at HGZ 1 in Aguascalientes, Villagrana Gutiérrez and Machuca Loeza (2023) found that 65.3 % of patients with CVD are women and 34.7 % are men.7 % corresponds to men, unlike our study where we found that the sex of greater predisposition are men, but in another study of the same university, now in the HGZ 2 Aguascalientes, Aguilar Soto and Ornelas Segovia (2023), also found women in 58%, This is due to endothelial dysfunction triggered by an inflammatory cascade of prothrombotic factors and vasoconstriction after menopause, since the endothelium is sensitive to the vasodilator properties of oestrogens, and when these levels decrease over time, there is arterial stiffness and atherosclerotic disease, increasing cardiovascular risk in women.According to the World Health Organisation, it is the second leading cause of death in the population over 60 years of age, with a worldwide prevalence in people aged 55 to 65 years of 11% and increasing to 22% between 65 and 69 years, 28% between 70 and 74 years. years, 32% between 75 and 79 years, 40% between 80 and 85 years and 43% over 85 years (González Piña and Landinez Martínez, 2016).Villagrana Gutiérrez and Machuca Loeza (2023), found that the mean age of presentation in women is around 63.80 years and in men around 63.80 years. men 62.87 years, results that coincide with our study, as the most frequent age of presentation was around the sixth decade of life. González Piña and Landinez Martínez (2016) in an applied prevalence survey in patients older than 65 years showed rates ranging from 65 to 91 per 1 000 inhabitants and their INTERSTROKE clinical trial, observed that there are 10 vascular risk factors where arterial hypertension, smoking, waist-to-hip ratio, unhealthy diet, physical inactivity, diabetes mellitus, alcohol consumption, psychosocial stress, cardiac pathology and apolipoprotein B/A1 ratio are responsible for approximately 90% of the total risk of CVD cases. Figueroa Casanova et al. (2022), in their descriptive study found hypertension to be 68.42%, followed by smoking with 34.21% and in third place dyslipidaemia and atrial fibrillation with 28.94%. In the same study, they found that in the United States, hypertension, smoking and alcoholism were found to be the main risk factors, which coincide with those found in this study, in which hypertension was the main risk factor.All patients who came to the hospital where the present study was conducted with a probable CVE were classified in the triage area, where the Cincinnati prehospital scale was used, being positive in all patients, corroborating that the weakness of the face, arms and speech difficulty can be assessed with high reliability by the patient himself, family, medical staff and nurses. When using the NIHSS scale, we found that the highest frequency of scores corresponds to Moderate Severe CSE, where the greatest neurological deterioration occurred on the third day, with the first patient leaving the study due to death; based on the data collected, it is important to emphasise surveillance and re-evaluation at 72 hours, as great similarity was found with another cross-sectional descriptive study, where Ali Khan et al., (2022), included 400 patients classified for CVD by NIHSS assessment, finding moderate CVD in 49% of cases, severe in 29% and mild in 22%. In this study, in the medical literature and other studies conducted, changes of ischaemic rather than haemorrhagic origin were observed in the cranial tomography; in a low percentage there may be neurological alteration without generating structural changes in the imaging study, these symptoms may reverse within a few hours of the event, without causing sequelae as in transient ischaemic attack, as reported in a retrospective study conducted at the University of Abuja Hospital, Kolade Yunusa et al, (2020), where 148 patients had tomographic findings compatible with ischaemic CVA in 56.1%, 41.2% haemorrhagic and 2.7% with normal findings; in another retrospective cross-sectional study, Edzie, et al., (2021), with 1 750 patients with CVA, where 1 237 (70.7%) represent CVA of ischaemic origin and 513 (29.3%) CVA of haemorrhagic origin. When performing the ASPECT scale during the evaluation of the cranial tomography, we mostly found a score of elimination for administering fibrinolytic treatment in agreement with a retrospective cohort study, Almallouhi et al, (2021), which included a total of 2 345 patients who, when applying the ASPECT scale, found that the greater the involvement of brain areas, the greater the neurological alteration and the greater the sequelae with a high degree of physical dependency, finding that 2 132 patients (90.9%) had ASPECT, and 213 patients (9.1%) had an ASPECT of 2-5. Specifically in the time of care, according to the immediate arrival of each patient; the time that elapses from the patient's arrival in the emergency room to the administration of the appropriate treatment (known as door-to-needle time) is crucial for the management of CVE. In our study, none of the patients arrived in the indicated time, which is why it is a priority to carry out health promotion actions at the first level of care, identification and control of cardiovascular risk factors, timely detection of signs and symptoms of CVD, with the goal of early identification of the risk of CVD and that on arrival of a patient at the different levels of medical care, treatment with intravenous fibrinolytic therapy is given in at least 10% of patients with CVD; Once this care protocol is implemented in the Hospital General de Zona 32 in Minatitlán, Veracruz, it will be gradually achieved that 100% of patients will comply with the stipulations of the PAI Brain Code algorithm (2022). In the emergency department, care was generally provided by the general practitioner, where it was found that there is a delay in the recognition of symptoms suggestive of CVE, due to the high demand of patients requesting care and the short time allocated to each patient; the emergency physician is dedicated to hospitalised patients with serious diagnoses. In addition, a brief evaluation of the Cincinnati scale and no application of the NIHSS scale was performed; In an observational, descriptive, cross-sectional, retrospective, retrospective study of the electronic clinical record of patients with CVE in the emergency department, Aguilar Soto and Ornelas Segovia, (2023), analysed compliance with the recommendations of the medical approach to patients with CVE where a significant difference was observed in the category of emergency physician who applied both scales compared with the other category in which the general practitioner, family physician and internist are grouped. When analysing medical and nursing care times, we found that according to the average time, there are patients who can be left outside treatment window, just by waiting for care, which represents a greater risk of complications, since the taking of vital signs, the assessment of a permeable airway, a lack of peripheral access are delayed for haemodynamic and respiratory stabilisation, being reflected in greater number of sequelae, which limit or hinder the quality of life in the patient with neurological damage; In a non-probabilistic study by convenience, Villagrana Gutiérrez and Machuca Loeza, (2023), also observed that there are factors that can delay the time in the administration of treatment, such as technical problems, delayed test results and incorrect assessment by emergency personnel, finding similarities with our study. All patients underwent simple cranial tomography, however, the time taken to perform the imaging study meant that our patients were not candidates for fibrinolytic treatment, as there was no tomograph in the unit and additional time of approximately 30 minutes was required to transfer the patient to another unit for the tomography. Therefore, time and the lack of a CT scanner in the unit have been the main factors related to the interruption and non-adherence to the algorithm. Aguilar

Soto and Ornelas Segovia, (2023) confirmed in their study that it took 45 minutes to perform the CT scan and 53 minutes to perform the fibrinolysis. This differs from the first 25 minutes from patient admission to the emergency department established in PAI Código cerebro, (2022), which also specifies that fibrinolytic therapy should be analysed within the first 20 minutes after performing fibrinolysis. the skull CT scan or within 3 to 4.5 hours of symptom onset. With regard to the adjuvant treatment of CVE, and specifically in relation to the control and management arterial hypertension, a delay was observed in the time taken to start pharmacological treatment, in addition to the fact that according to the PAI algorithm, code brain, (2022) the drugs of first choice corresponding to hydralazine, nitroprusside and labetalol are not used, Both the general practitioner and specialists used other antihypertensive drugs to control blood pressure, and dual antiplatelet therapy was used in a low percentage. It was also found that there was a significant discrepancy in the time of assessment of the specialties, which could have influenced the clinical evolution of each patient and the clinical, diagnostic and treatment congruence. According to the PAI Brain Code (2022), the patients in the present study were not within the window for the administration of thrombolysis, as there are several factors that can delay the time from admission to imaging, as was found in a hospital in Arequipa, Peru, by Cueva Bustos and Pérez Corrales (2023), where they determined the relationship between the time of illness and initiation of treatment in patients with CVE. There are also other factors that influence this association, such as hospital infrastructure and accessibility to thrombolysis, the number of physicians in the emergency department and trained health personnel.

In another descriptive observational multicentre cross-sectional observational study, Figueroa Casanova et al., (2022), evaluated the clinical outcomes of acute management with thrombolysis in patients who presented with ischaemic CVEs in two institutions.In association with our study, in the future, the modification of the algorithm times could be implemented in our hospital, taking into account its infrastructural resources, and thus include a greater number of patients who are candidates for thrombolysis, with the certainty that a satisfactory result will be obtained in the clinical evolution of the patients. We found that the sequelae presented after CVE are similar to other studies which found that language impairment, facial asymmetry, hemiplegia and aphasia were common symptoms in this population (Villagrana Gutiérrez and Machuca Loeza, 2023) hence the importance of surveillance and prevention in all adult ages since, according to the degree of neurological impairment, will be the severity of CVE, it is estimated that deaths and disability from this disease will more than double by 2030 (Figueroa Casanova et al., 2022). In the follow-up of the improvement of the sequelae, in two of the subgroups of the sample it was not possible to corroborate the clinical evolution, as there was a loss of follow-up bias, in the rest the clinical evolution was verified, similar to a study by Figueroa Casanova et al. (2022), where the review of consultation notes from other specialties such as internal medicine and cardiology was made, in our case the follow-up with internal medicine, neurology, neurosurgery and physical medicine and rehabilitation was verified. Physical and functional dependence is found in a high percentage in our study, however, the clinical evolution of the patient in a period of 3 months was found to be favoured by the effects of physical therapy and rehabilitation, because it has a neuromodulatory effect on the nerve pathways, as mentioned by Bardales Ayarza and Risco Glaston, (2023). At At the same time, we observed that patients with a high score on the NIHSS scale have a torpid evolution at hospital discharge, even with a high risk of death, this includes patients who did not receive and who received treatment with fibrinolysis; Figueroa Casanova et al, (2022) report in their study on the management of ischaemic CVE with fibrinolytic therapy where they found that patients with NIHSS scale at admission had a mean of 17.63 points (SD 3.92; p=

0.008) in patients who died at 90 days, compared to those who did not die who had a score at admission of 12.19 points (SD 4.97). In this follow-up, we corroborated that the sequelae following CVE can limit functions and activities of daily living, affecting people's quality of life; studies that provide information on patients who have undergone thrombolysis and those who have not would provide a solid basis making decisions on health policies that improve the efficacy and safety of acute management of CVE.

CONCLUSION AND RECOMMENDATION

In this study it was found that there is no adherence to the PAI Brain Code algorithm, as patients are not involved in primary prevention and in recognising symptoms suggestive of CVE in order to go immediately to the emergency department. It is corroborated that the PAI Brain Code algorithm is not complied with, due to infrastructure, administrative reasons or lack of knowledge of the symptoms, which had a significant influence in this study so that no patient was in the therapeutic window for applying fibrinolytic therapy, directly affecting the quality of life of patients due to the high frequency of sequelae, affecting their physical independence; thus, continuous training on this guide would have satisfactory results for the personnel involved in the care of these patients.

REFERENCES

Aguilar, E., Rodríguez, G., García, K., Garfias, C., Hernández, E., and Oropeza, N. (2022). Acute Stroke Care in Mexico City: The Hospital Phase of a Stroke Surveillance Study. Brain sciences, 12, 1-10. **https://doi.org/10.3390/brainsci12070865**

Aguilar Soto, N. E. and Ornelas Segovia, R.O. (2023). Characterization of compliance with the guidelines for diagnosis and early treatment of ischemic cerebral vascular disease in the second and third level of care in the emergency department of the Hospital General de Zona No. 2, OOAD Aguascalientes [Specialty thesis, Universidad Autónoma de Aguascalientes].

http://hdl.handle.net/11317/2681

Ali Khan, M.S., Ahmad, S., Ghafoor, B., Haris Shah, M., Mumtaz, H., Ahmad, W., Banu, R., Ahmad, I., Iqbal, J., Muhammad Ismail Safi, M. and Khan, F. (2022). Inpatient assessment of the neurological outcome of acute stroke patients based on the National Institute of Health Stroke Scale (NIHSS). Annals Of Medicine And Surgery, 82, 1-5.

https://doi.org/10.1016/j.amsu.2022.104770

Almallouhi, E., Al Kasab, S., Hubbard, Z., Bass, E. C., Porto,G., Alawieh, A., Chalhoub, R., Jabbour, P.M., Starke, R.M., Wolfe, S.Q., Arthur, A.S., Samaniego, E., Maier, I., Howard, B.M., Rai, A., Park, M.S., Mascitelli, J., Psychogios, M., De Leacy, R., ... Dumont, T., Levitt, M.R., Polifka, A., Osbun, J., Crosa, R., Tae Kim, J., Casagrande, W., Yoshimura, S., Matouk, C., T Kan, P., W Williamson, R., Gory, B., Mokin, M., Fragata, I., Zaidat, O., Yoo, A.J. and Spiotta, A.M. (2021). Outcomes of Mechanical Thrombectomy for Patients with Stroke Presenting with Low Alberta Stroke Program Early

Computed Tomography Score in the Early and Extended Window. JAMA Network Open, 4(12), 1-12.

https://doi.org/10.1001/jamanetworkopen.2021.37708

Bao, Z., Zhang, Z., Zhou, G., Zhang, A., Shao, A., and Zhou, F. (2022). Novel mechanisms and therapeutic targets for ischemic stroke: A focus on gut Microbiota. Frontiers in Cellular Neuroscience, 16, 871720. https://doi.org/10.3389/fncel.2022.871720

Bardales Ayarza, G. L. and Risco Glaston, D.E. (2023). Impact factors of physical therapy and rehabilitation in the care of patients with sequelae of cerebrovascular disease in two national hospitals of Loreto year 2022-2023. [B.Sc. in Medical Technology. Specialty: Physical Therapy and Rehabilitation, Scientific University of Peru]. http://hdl.handle.net/20.500.14503/2614

Calero Moscoso, C. S. (2023). Diagnosis and Treatment of Acute Ischemic Cerebrovascular Disease (Stroke Code). CAMbios 22 (2), 1-17.

https://orcid.org/0000-0003-2070-0322

Choreño Parra, J.A., Carnalla Cortés, M. and Guadarrama Ortiz P. (2019). Medicina Interna from México. Ischemic cerebrovascular disease: extensive review of the literature for the first contact physician. 35(1):61- 79.

https://doi.org/10.24245/mim.v35i1.2212

Coronel, A., Andrés, P., Cabrera, C., Zamora, T. and Vargas, H. (2020). Intravenous thrombolysis in ischemic stroke: Experience in a Popayán hospital, Cauca. Acta Neurol Colomb, 36(1), 11-17. https://doi.org/10.22379/24224022272.

Cueva Bustos, A. S. and Pérez Corrales, M.A. (2023). Relación entre el tiempo de enfermedad e inicio de tratamiento en pacientes con accidente cerebrovascular isquémico, en el Hospital Nacional Carlos Alberto Seguín

Escobedo de Arequipa, enero a diciembre del 2022. [Medicine degree thesis, Universidad Católica de Santa María].

https://repositorio.ucsm.edu.pe/handle/20.500.12920/12559

Czap, A. L. and Sheth, S. A. (2021). Overview of imaging modalities in stroke. Neurology, 97(20 Suppl 2), S42-S51.
https://doi.org/10.1212/WNL.0000000000012794

Edzie, E. K., Dzefi Tettey, K., Gorleku, P., Tutu Amankwa, A., Idun, E., Brakohiapa, E. K., Cudjoe, O., Quarshie, F., Edzie, R. A. and Asemah, A. R. (2021). Evaluation of the Anatomical Locations of Stroke Events From Computed Tomography Scan Examinations in a Tertiary Facility in Ghana. Cureus, 13(3),1-13.

https://doi.org/10.7759/cureus.14097

Fernandes, L., Santos, D., Santos, M. and Rocha, N. P. (2022). How to improve emergency information systems to optimize the care of acute stroke. Procedia Computer Science, 196, 606-614.
https://doi.org/10.1016/j.procs.2021.12.055

Figueroa Casanova, R., Patiño Rodríguez, H.M., Téllez Villa, J.A., Torrado Varón, M.A., Figueroa Legarda, J.S. and Saavedra Henao, J.D. (2022). Experience in the management of ischemic stroke in two tertiary level centres in the city of Ibagué (Colombia) between 2019 and June 2020. Acta Neurológica Colombiana, 38 (1), 12-22.

https://doi.org/10.22379/24224022396

García González, A.C., Ángeles Velásquez, J., Díaz Greene, E.J. and Rodríguez Weber, FL (2022). Poor prognostic factors associated with cerebral vascular disease: retrospective study at Hospital Angeles Pedregal. Acta Médica Grupo Ángeles, 20(2), 157-162.

https://doi.org/10.35366/104277
González Piña, R. and Landinez Martínez, D. (2016). Epidemiology, etiology and classification of cerebral vascular disease. Archivos de Medicina, 16 (2), 495-507.

https://doi.org/10.30554/archmed.16.2.1726.2016
Hans, D. and Graeme, H. (2020). Primary and secondary prevention of ischemic stroke and cerebral hemorrhage. JACC focus seminar, 75(15), 1804- 1818. https://doi.org/10.1016/j.jacc.2019.12.072
Jurcau, A., & Simion, A. (2021). Neuroinflammation in cerebral ischemia and ischemia/reperfusion injuries: From pathophysiology to therapeutic strategies. International Journal of Molecular Sciences, 23(1), 14. https://doi.org/10.3390/ijms23010014
Mexican Social Security Institute, based on Article 83 of the Mexican Social Security Law.

L.F.D.A. in relation to Article 46 of the R.L.F.D.A. (12 January 2022). Comprehensive Care Protocols - Cardiovascular Diseases - Brain Code. www.imss.gob.mx/sites/all/statics/profesionalesSalud/investigacionSal ud/historical/programs/05-pai-codigo-cerebrohttps://.pdf
Kolade Yunusa H. O., Adamu Yaro I. and Yusuf, L. (2020). Cranial computed tomography imaging of patients with stroke in a tertiary facility. West African Journal of Radiology, 27 (1), 46-51.

https://doi.org/10.4103/wajr.wajr_2_19
López Tapia, J.D., Sandoval Mussi, A.Y., Cuéllar Rodríguez, E., Umaña Ramírez, M.V., García, D.E., Montes, M., Laica Sailema, N.R., López Terán, G.P., Grajales, D., Uribe Moya, S.E., Irrizarri, Y., Sánchez Arreola, L. D., Sandoval Mosqueda, L.E., Saavedra Uribe, J. and Obregón Mendoza,

M.G. (2022). Latin American consensus of cerebral vascular event of the Latin American Federation of Emergency Medicine (FLAME).

Journal of Education and Research in Emergencies, 4(3), 213- 247.
https://doi.org/10.24875/reie.22000083

Man, J., Sol, D. and Kim, M. (2021). Hemorrhagic transformation after ischemic stroke: Mechanisms and management. Front Neurol, 12, 1-12.
https://doi.org/10.3389/fneur.2021.703258

Mohamed, G. A., Marmarchi, F., Fonkeu, Y., Alshaer, Q., Rangaraju, S., Carr, M., Jones, A., Peczka, M., Contreras, I., Bahdsalvi, L., Brasher, C., and Nahab, F. (2022). Cincinnati Prehospital Stroke Scale Implementation of an Urban County Severity-Based Stroke Triage Protocol: Impact and Outcomes on a Comprehensive Stroke Center. Journal of stroke and cerebrovascular diseases, 31 (8), 1-6.

https://doi.org/10.1016/j.jstrokecerebrovasdis.2022.106575

Nogles T. and Galuska M. 2022. Middle Cerebral Artery Stroke.statpearls. 1-11.
https://europepmc.org/books/n/statpearls/article-

25121/?extid=29262225&src=med

Phipps, M. S and Cronin, C. A (2020). Management of acute ischemic stroke The BMJ, 1- 21.

https://doi.org/10.1136/bmj.l6983

Pineda Sanabria, J. P. and Tolosa Cubillos, J. M. (2022). Ischaemic stroke of the middle cerebral artery. Revista Repertorio De Medicina Y Cirugía, 31(1), 20-32.
https://doi.org/10.31260/RepertMedCir.01217372.1104

Rais, K., Mansour, A. and Ulvi, B. (2022). MicroRNA: An emerging predictive, diagnostic, prognostic and therapeutic strategy in ischaemic stroke. Cell Mol Neurobiol, 42(5), 1301-1319.
https://doi.org/10.1007/s10571-020-01028-5

Romero, I., Guzman, A. and Islas, F. (2018). Successful thrombolysis in

cerebrovascular disease: a case report. Rev Sanid Milit Mex, 72(5-6), 359-362.
www.scielo.org.mx/pdf/rsm/v72n5-6/0301-696X-rsm-72-5-6-359.pdf

https://Saini, V., Guada, L. and Yavagal, D. R. (2021). Global epidemiology of stroke. and access to acute ischemic stroke interventions. Neurology, 97(20 Suppl 2), S6-S16.
https://doi.org/10.1212/WNL.0000000000012781

Solorio, J., Saldana, M., Lytras, M., Moreno, M. and Yáñez, C. (2021). Brain Hemorrhage classification in CT scan images using Minimalist Machine Learning. Diagnostics, 11, 1-37.

Teleb, M. S., Ver Hage, A., Carter, J., Jayaraman, M. V. and McTaggart, R. A. (2017). Stroke vision, aphasia, neglect (VAN) assessment-a novel emergent large vessel occlusion screening tool: pilot study and comparison with current clinical severity indices. Journal of Neurointerventional Surgery, 9(2), 122-126.
https://doi.org/10.1136/neurintsurg-2015-012131

Tuna, M. A. and Rothwell, P. P. (2021). Diagnosis of non-consensus transient ischaemic attacks with focal, negative, and non-progressive symptoms: population-based validation by investigation and prognosis. Lancet, 397 (10277), 902-912.

https://doi.org/10.1016/s0140-6736(20)31961-9

Villagrana Gutiérrez, G. L. and Machuca Loeza, M.L. (2023). Needle door time in patients with ischaemic cerebral vascular event older than
20 years attended in the adult emergency department of HGZ 1, Aguascalientes [Specialty thesis, Universidad Autónoma de Aguascalientes].

http://hdl.handle.net/11317/2705

Xu, J., Zhang, Y. and Nie, G. (2021). Intelligent antithrombotic nanomedicines: Progress, opportunities, and challenges. View (Beijing, China), 2(2), 20200145.

https://doi.org/10.1002/viw.20200145

AUTHOR BIOGRAPHY

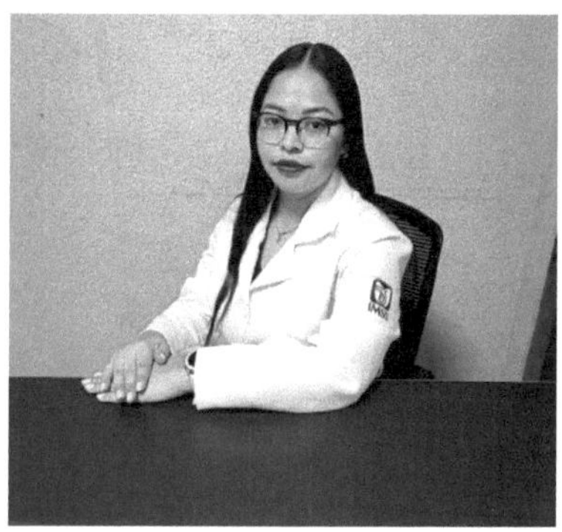

Born 08 November 1986. Native and resident of the city of Acayucan, Veracruz. Graduated with a degree in Medicine from the Universidad Autónoma de Veracruz Villa Rica, Veracruz campus; Specialist in Family Medicine at the Hospital General de Zona N° 32 Minatitlán of the Instituto Mexicano del Seguro Social (Mexican Social Security Institute).

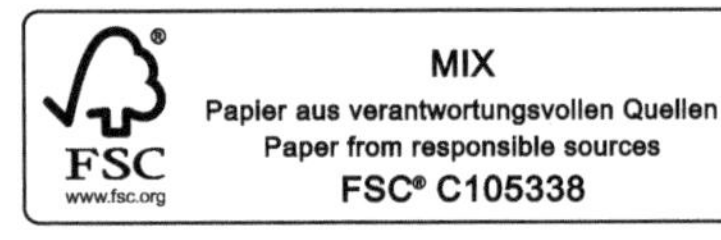

Printed by Books on Demand GmbH, Norderstedt / Germany